This book is a full yoga class that parent and child can experience together simply by following the instructions and illustrations. The sequence incorporates all the benefits of yoga including meditation, cardiovascular conditioning, relaxation, and breathing techniques. The class is designed to motivate children to be active, build confidence, and manage the spectrum of emotions that they experience in their day-to-day activities-- basically stress management for kids!

Dedicated to Max, Da Da, and Gi

Sit in a comfortable seated position. You have many options.

Criss-Cross Applesauce

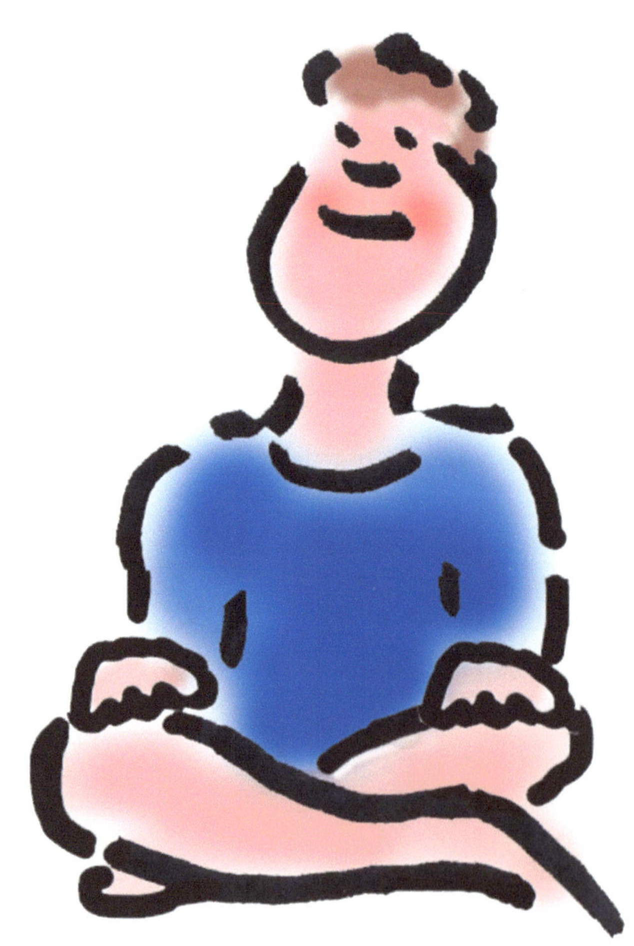

or Half Lotus

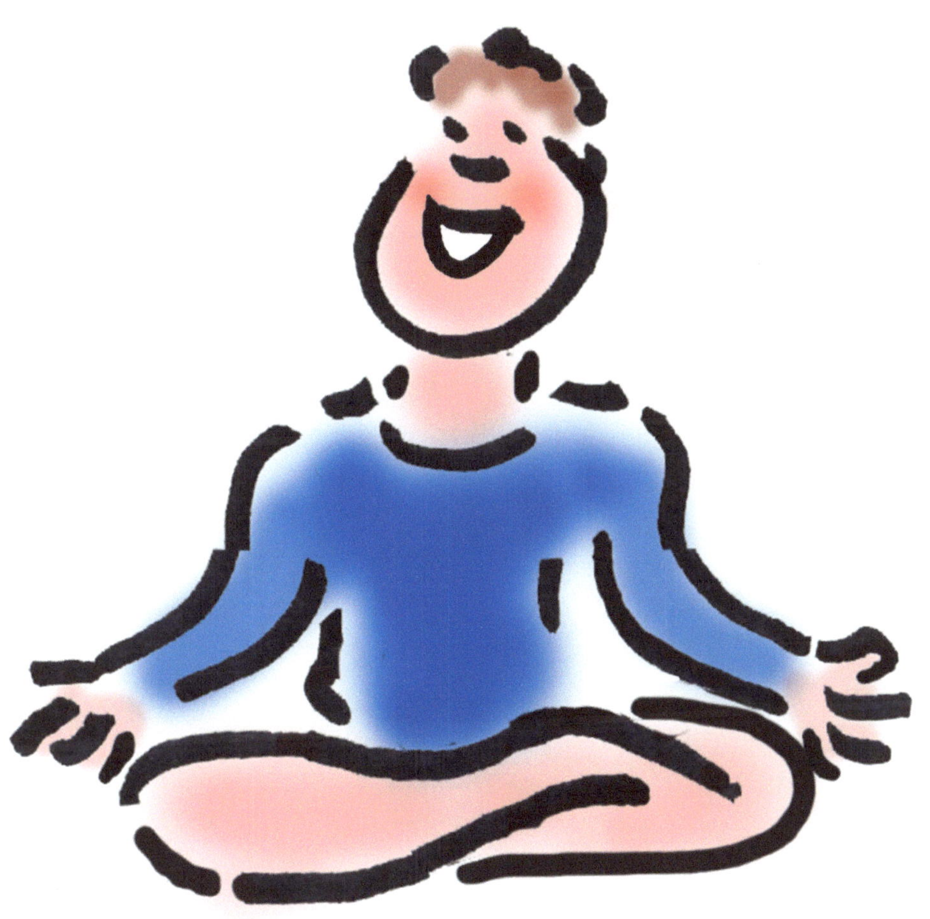

or Full Lotus

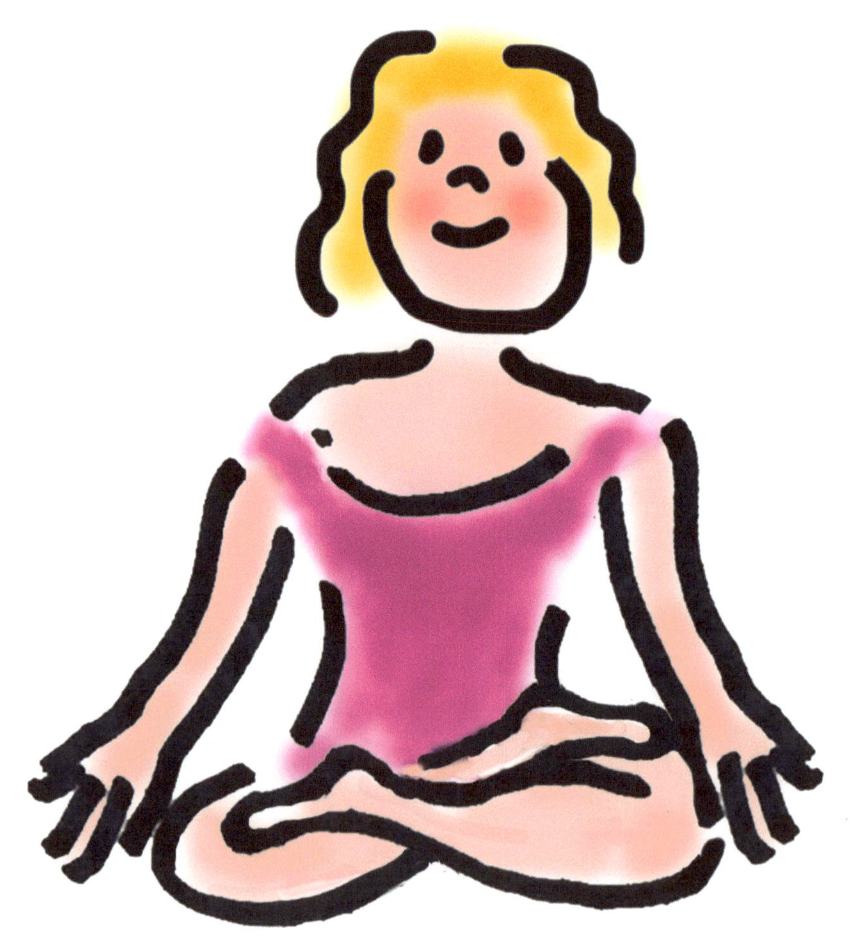

or really however you want

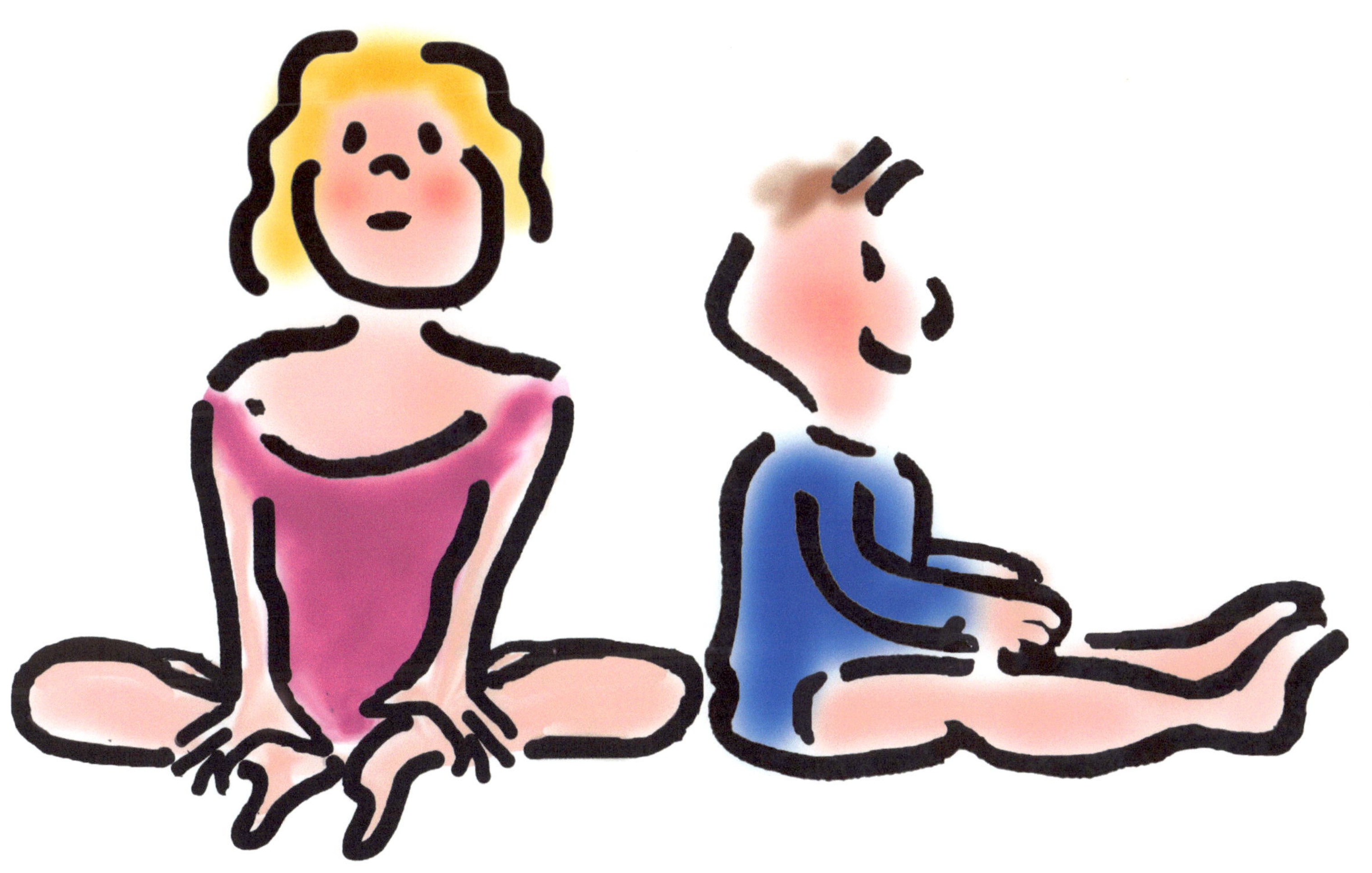

Take a deep breath and say
"ommm."

Pound your chest and yell it like Tarzan.

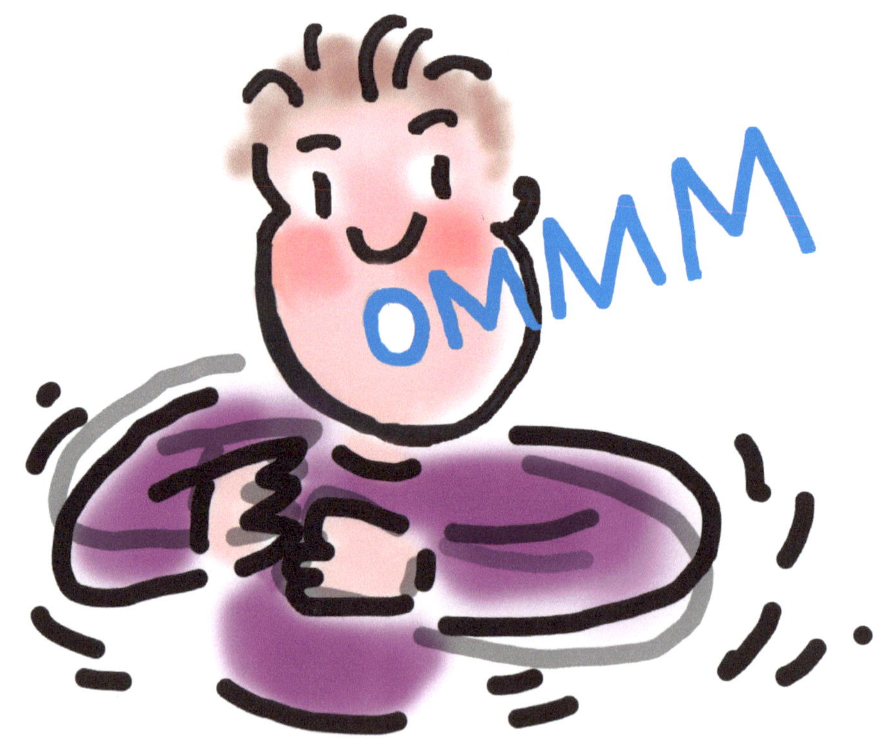

Pretend you are underwater and say:

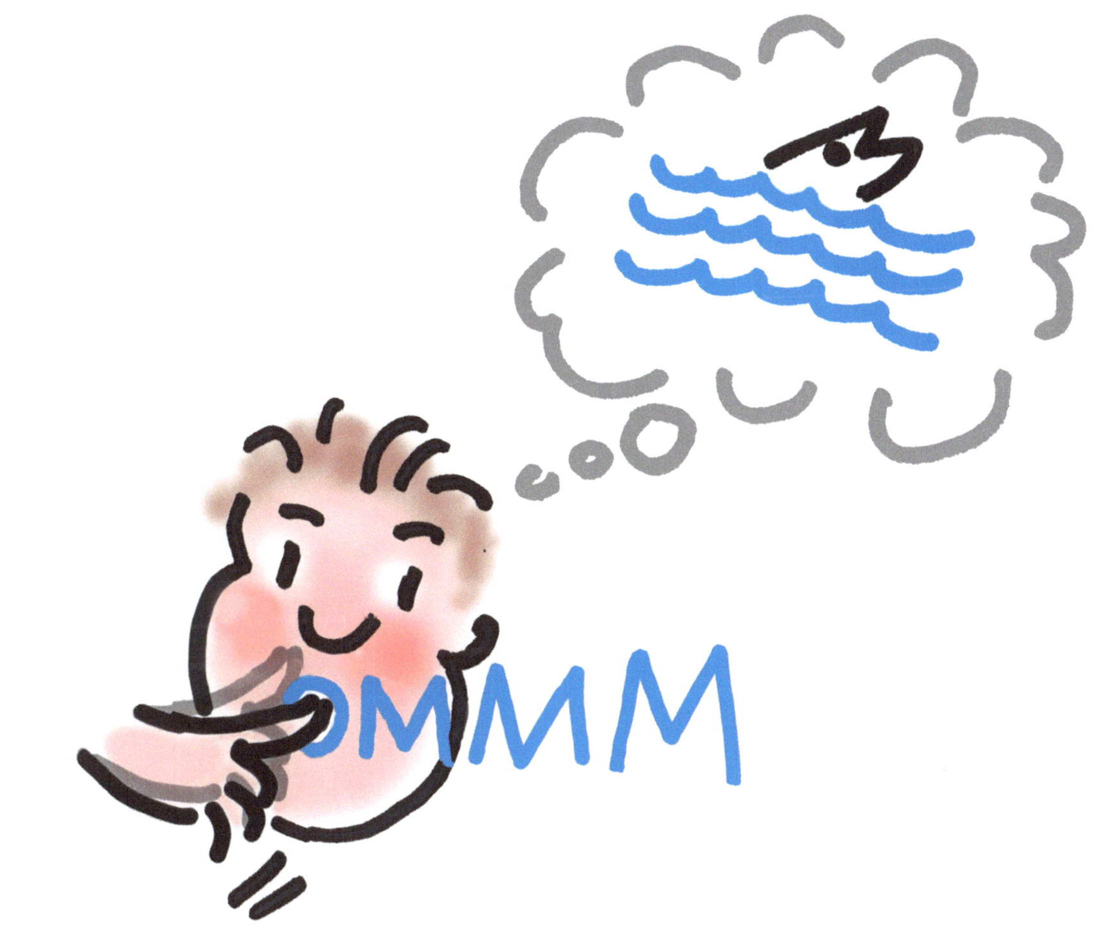

Say it one more time in a serious manner.

Put on your
yoga glasses.

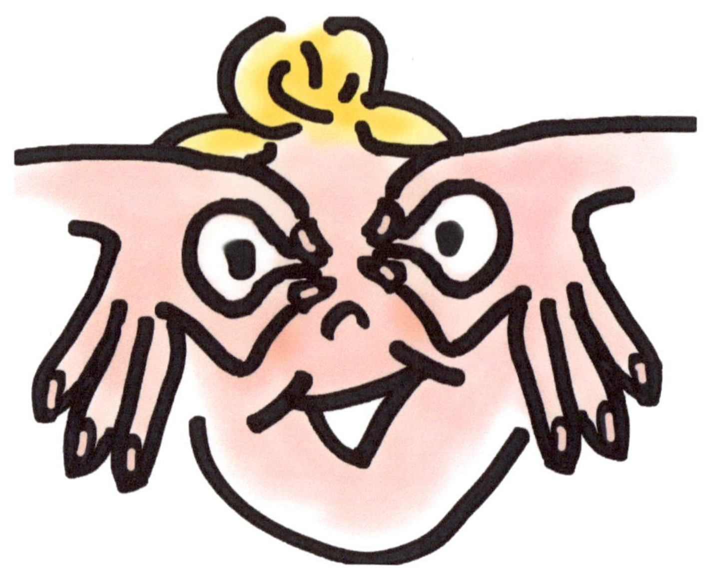

Place your yoga
glasses on your
knees.

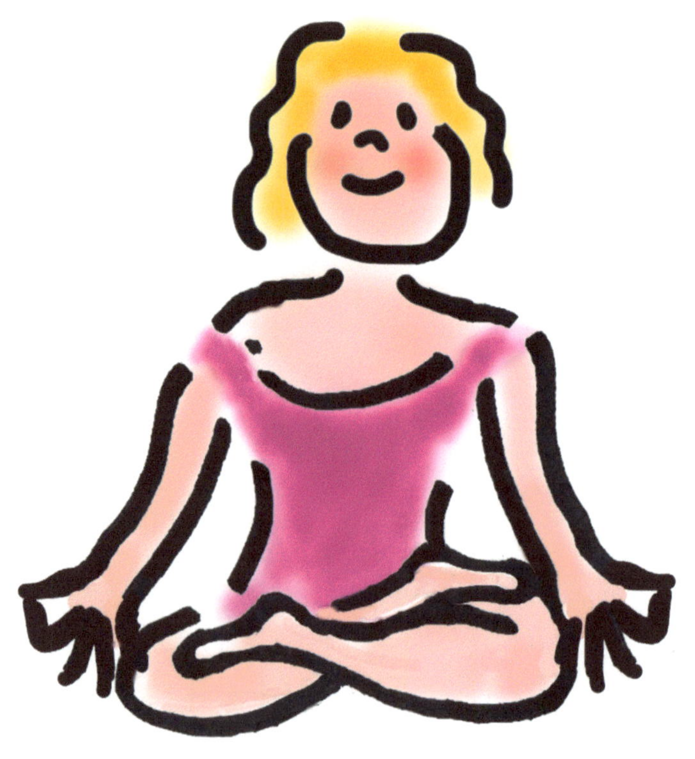

As you touch each finger
to your thumb, say:

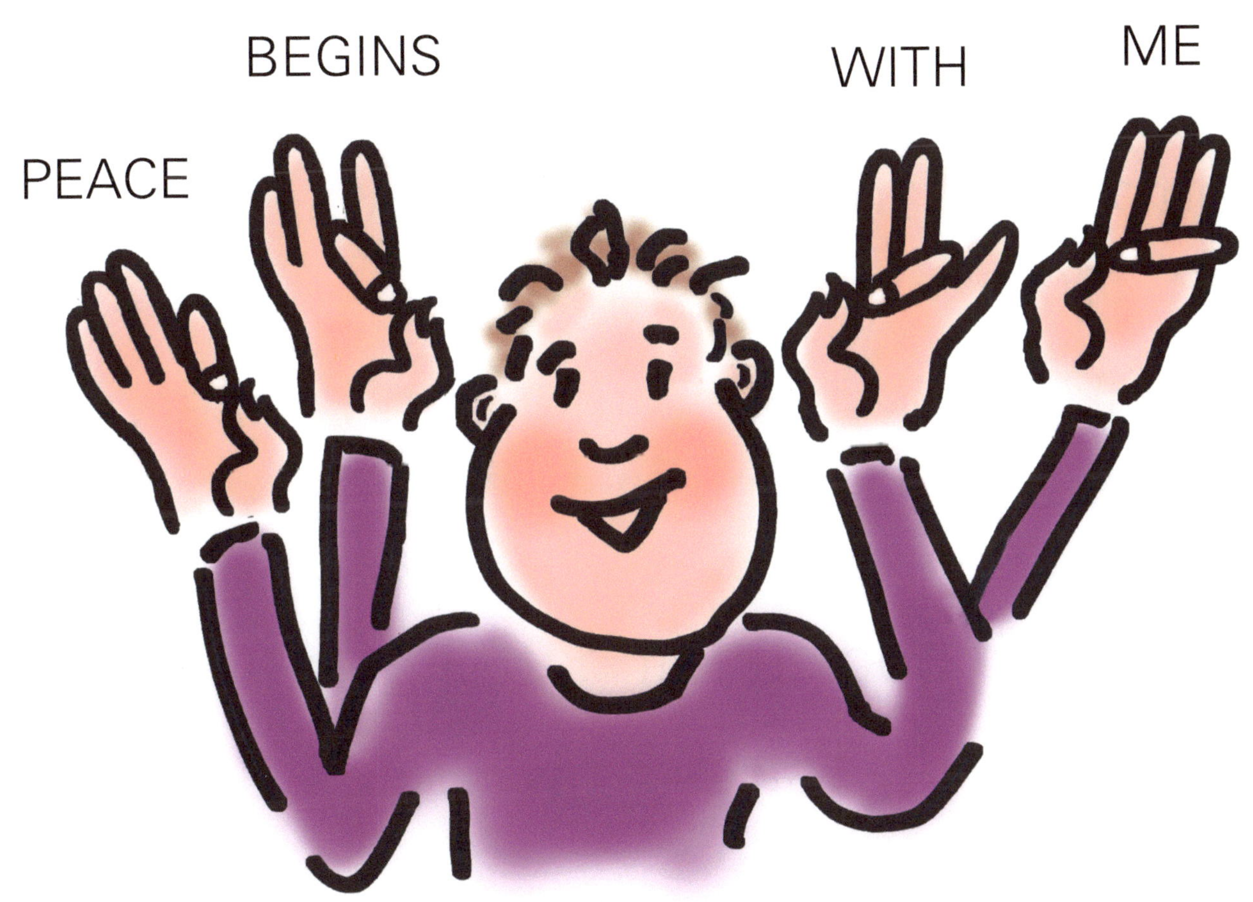

Repeat this phrase quieter each time
until you can only hear it in your head.

Warm up like animals.

A long time ago, humans would spend a lot of time sitting-- days, weeks, months just sitting. And they noticed that their arms started to hurt and their legs and their tushies too.

They took a look around them and observed the movements of animals like cats, cows, and cobras. Once they started moving like animals, their bodies felt better.

Let's warm up like these animals.

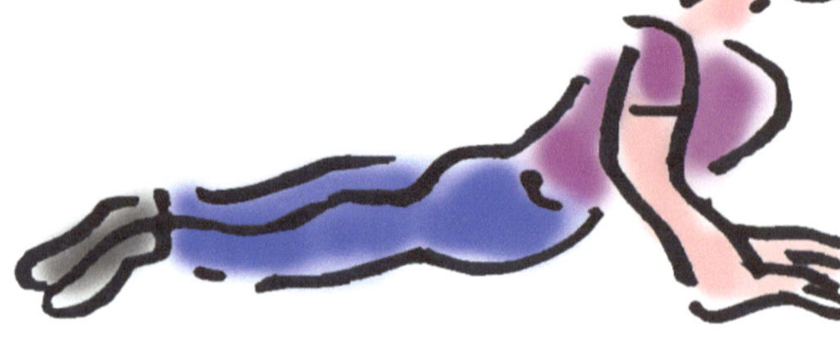

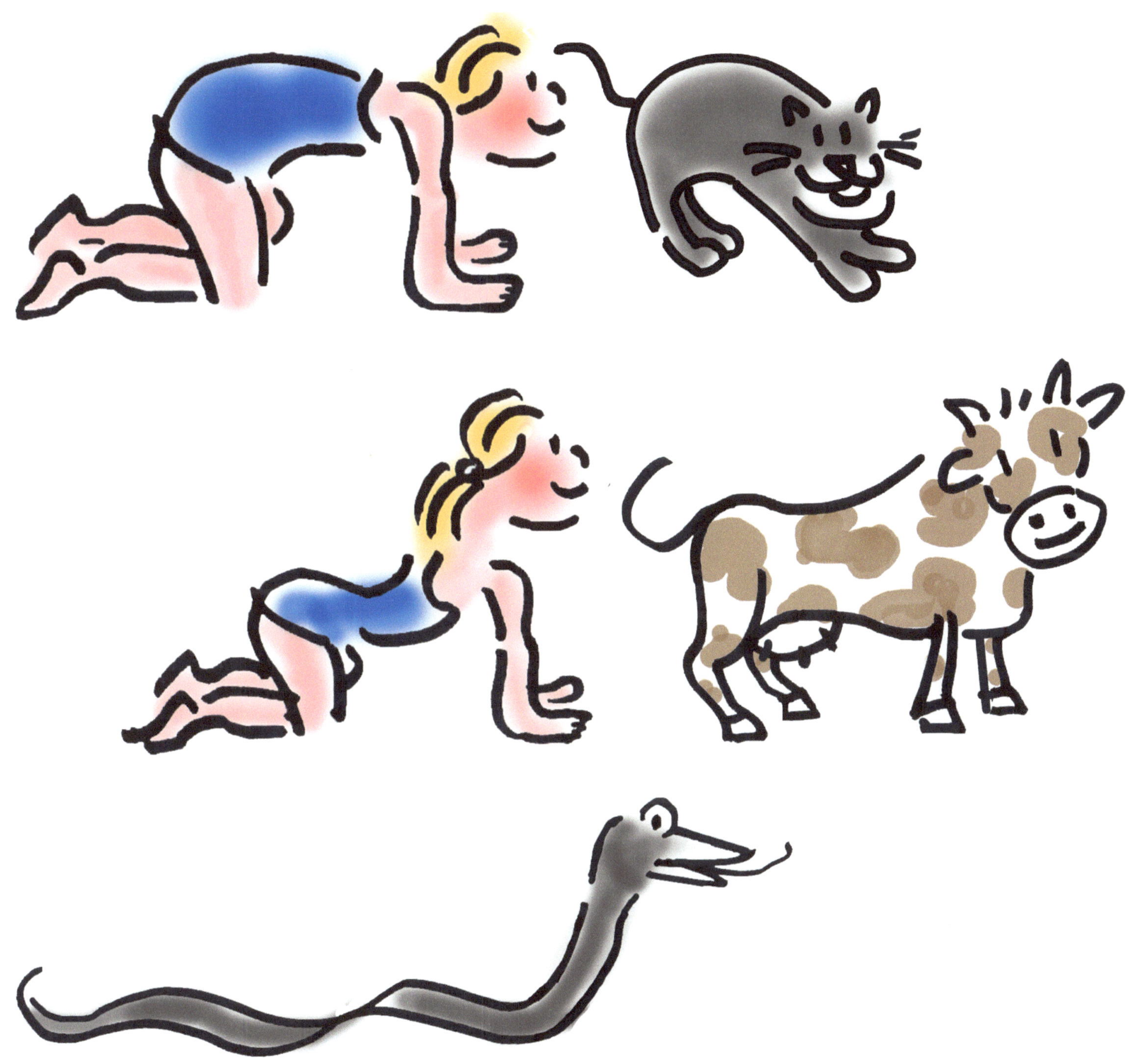

Energize with pretend pizza.

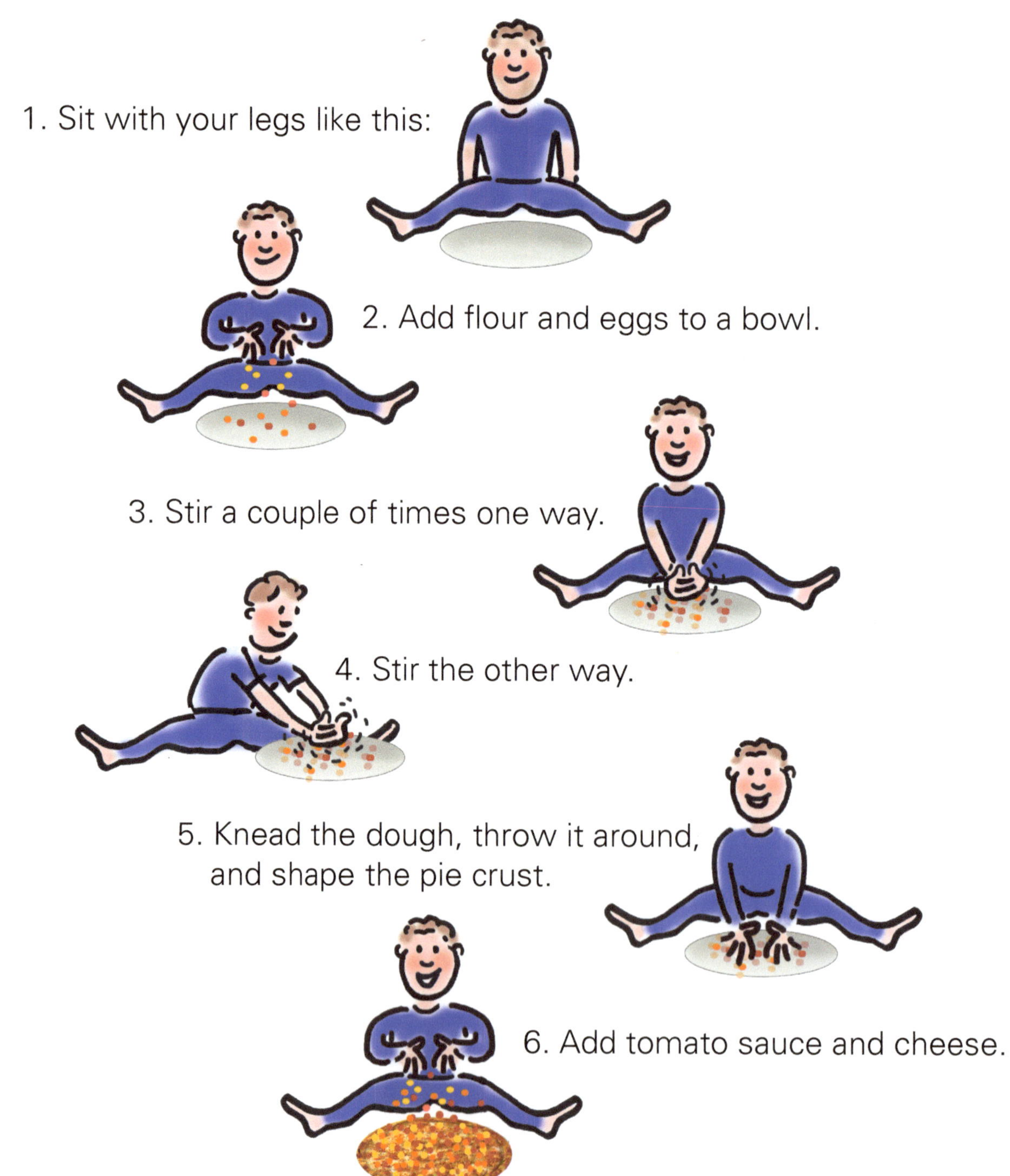

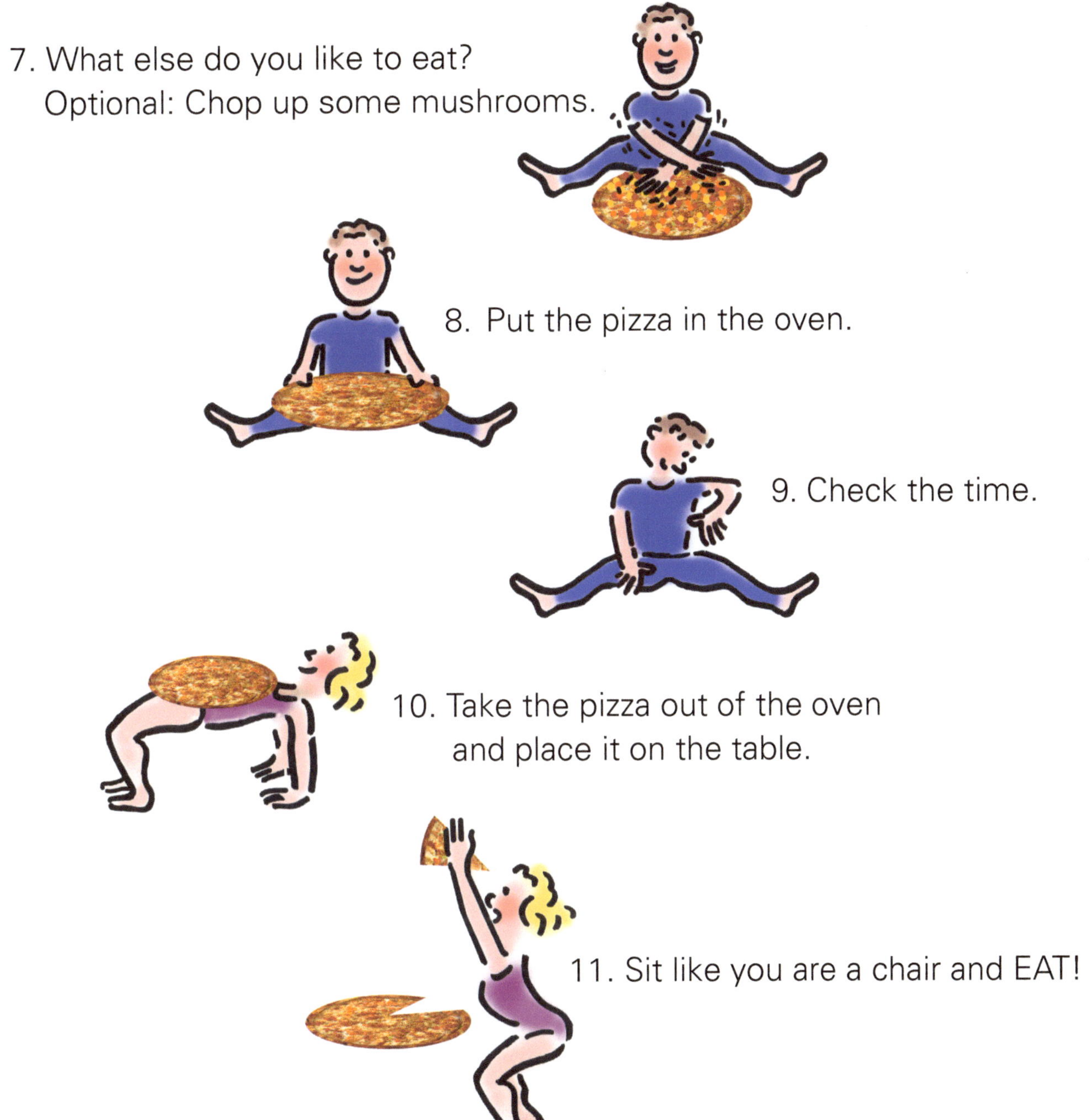

7. What else do you like to eat?
    Optional: Chop up some mushrooms.

8. Put the pizza in the oven.

9. Check the time.

10. Take the pizza out of the oven
     and place it on the table.

11. Sit like you are a chair and EAT!

Repeat after me to do a sun salutation.

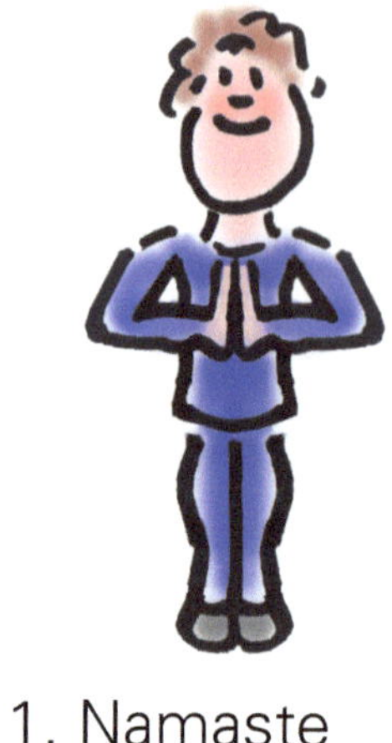

1. Namaste

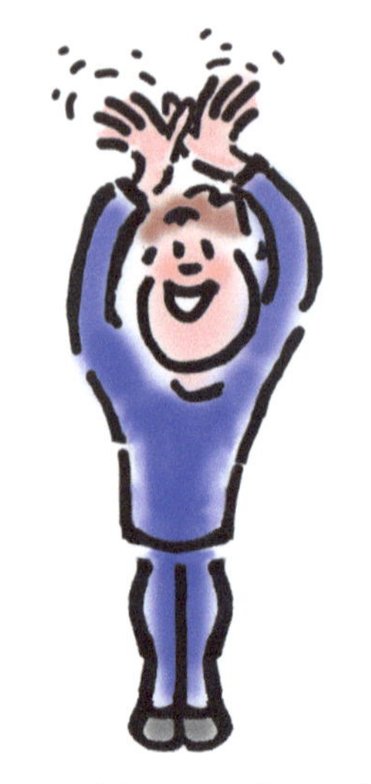

12. Butterfly Up

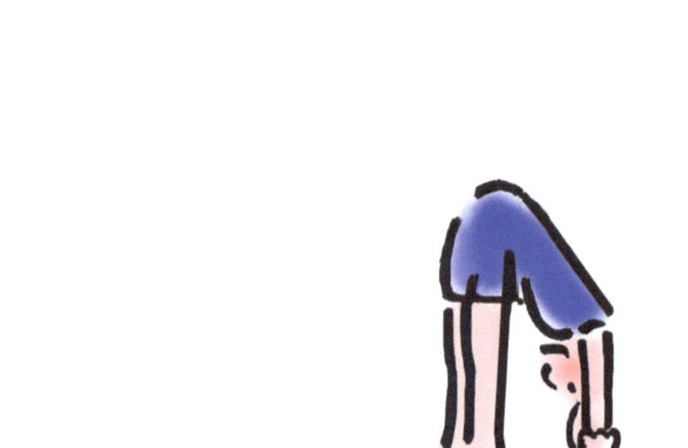

11. Ragdoll

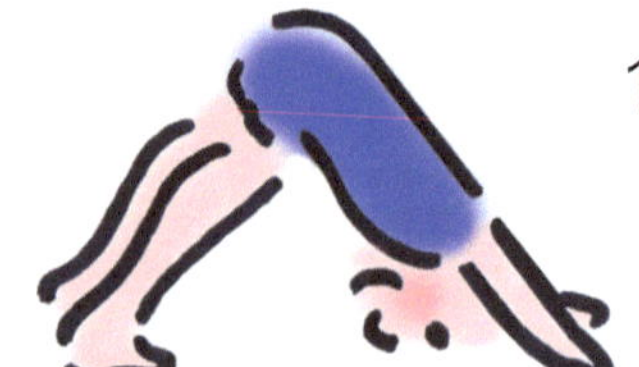

10. Downward Dog

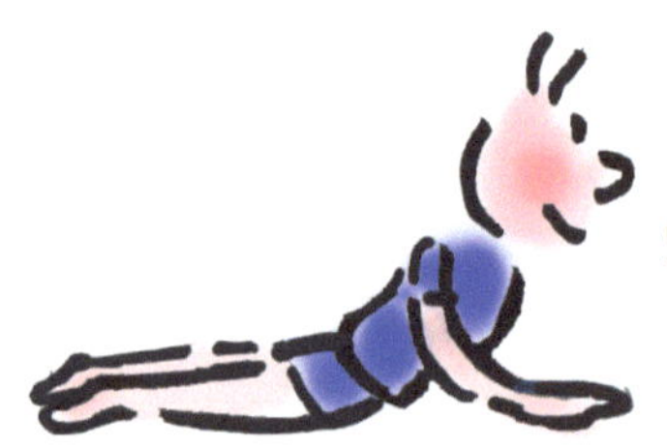

9. Upward Ah Woooooo

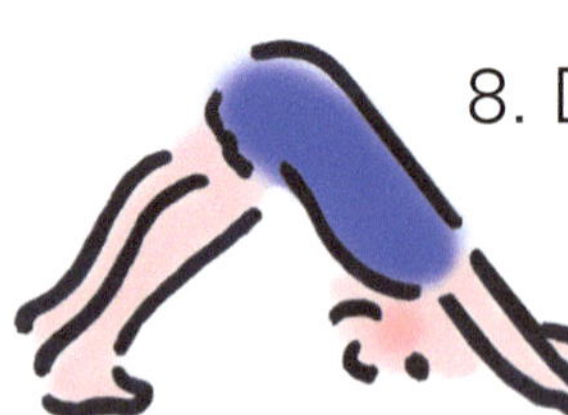

8. Downward Woof

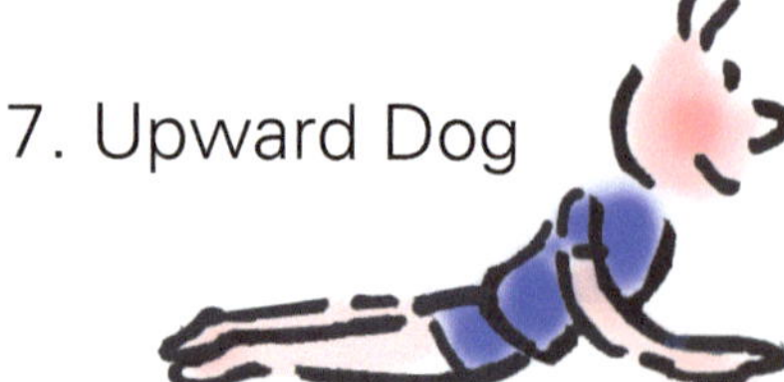

7. Upward Dog

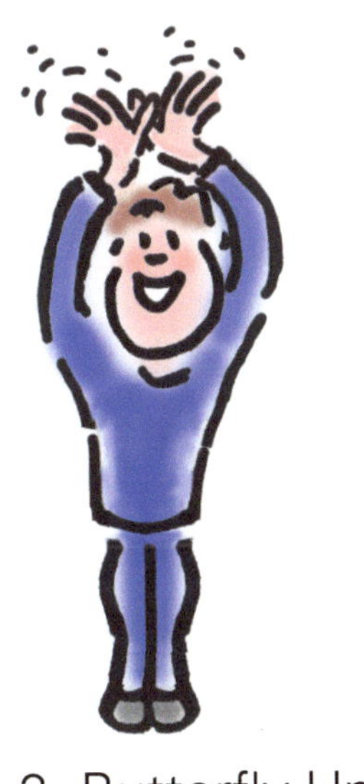

2. Butterfly Up

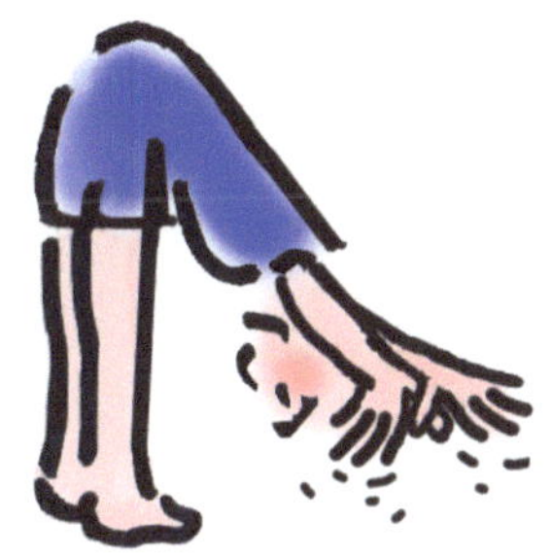

3. Butterfly Down

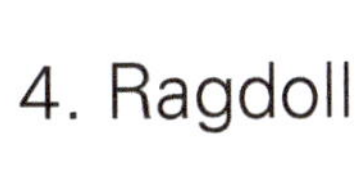

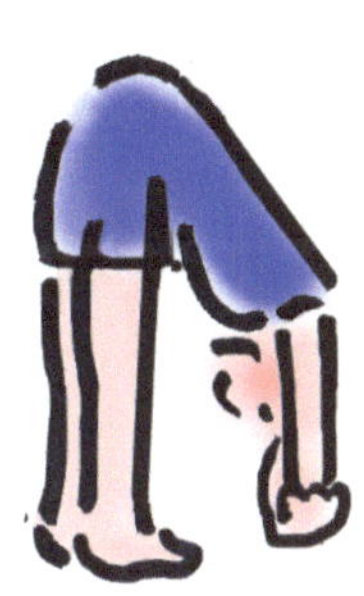

4. Ragdoll

5. Plank Pose

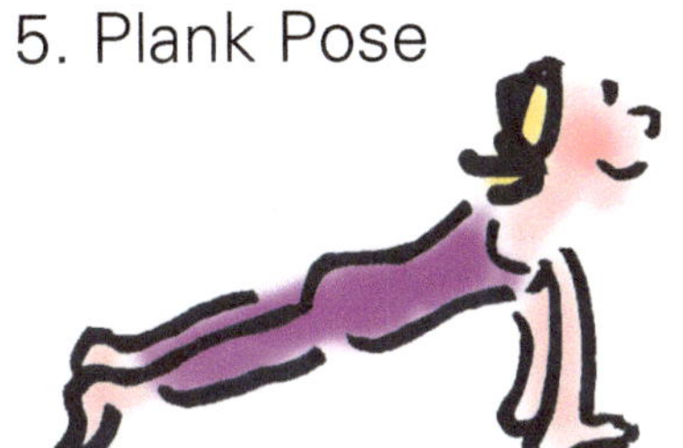

6. Downward Dog

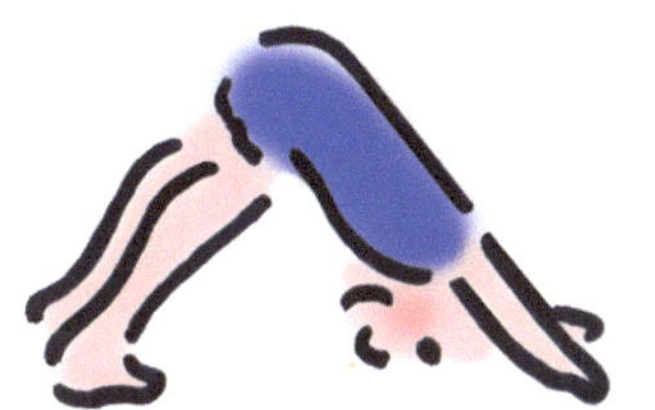

Let's do it again!

Balance like a tree.

Shift your weight to one foot. Place the other foot on your calf. Pretend your arms are branches swaying in the wind. Repeat on the other side.

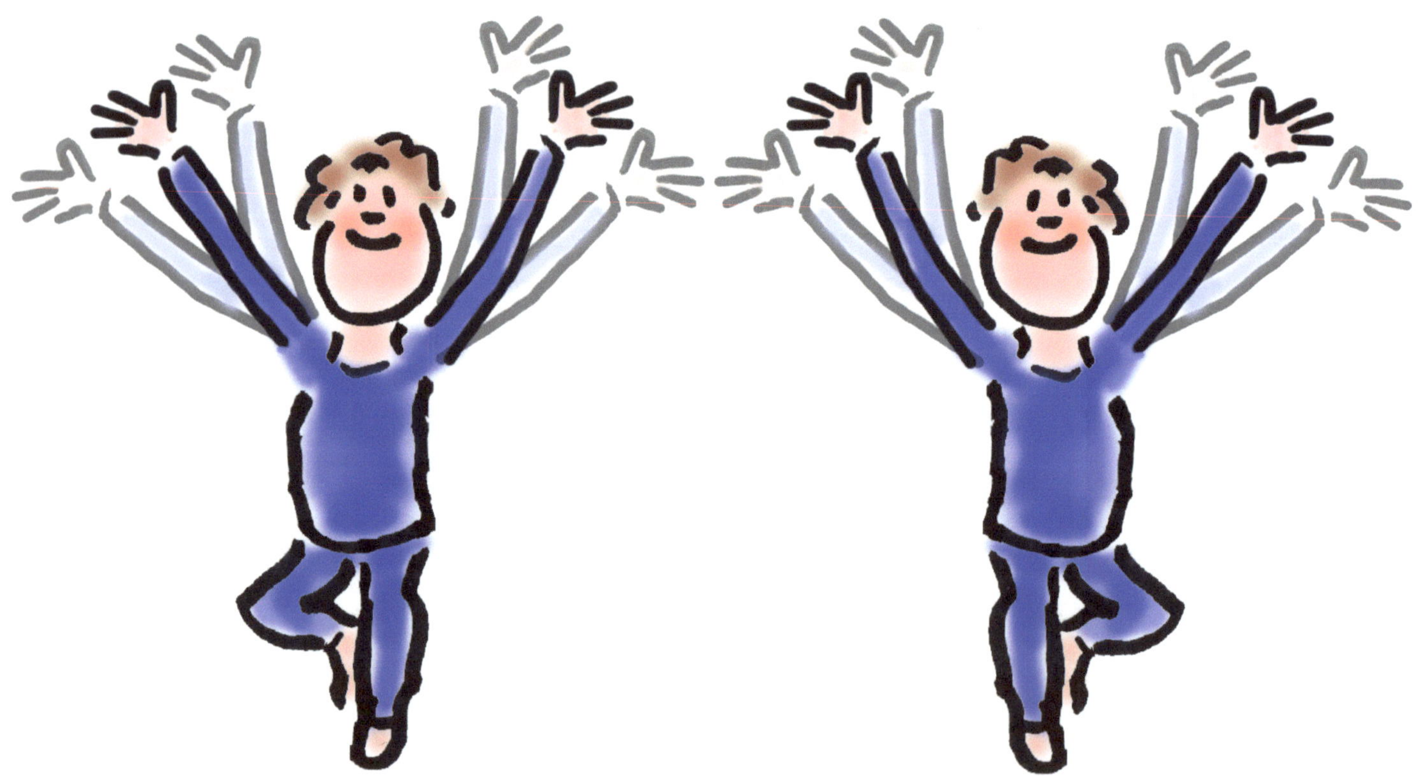

Remember that what you do to one side you must do to the other in tree pose and every pose.

Great job!

Celebrate the sun salutation and balancing pose you just did by throwing pom poms in the air! Use real ones or cotton balls if you have them. Can you pick some up with your toes? Can you move one across the room by blowing on it? Remember to clean them up.

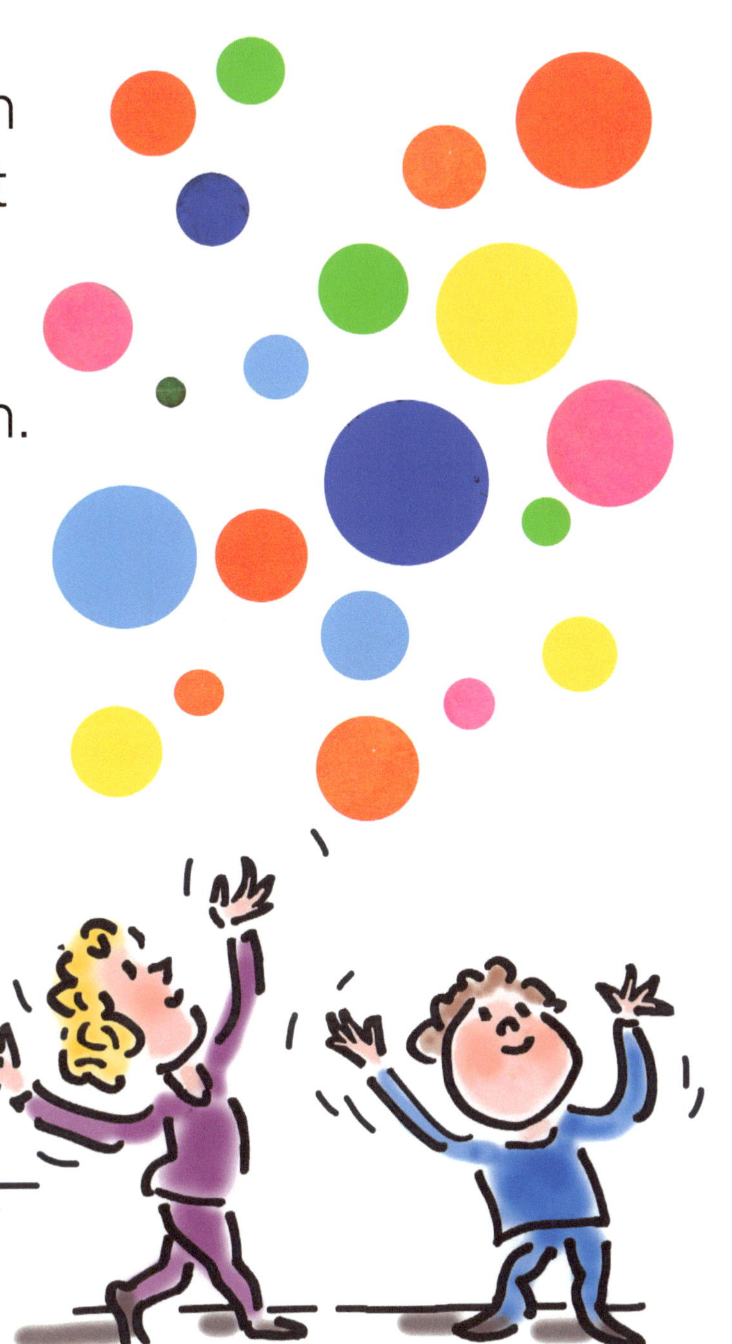

Go upside down.

Put your legs up the wall.
You may need a grown-up to help.

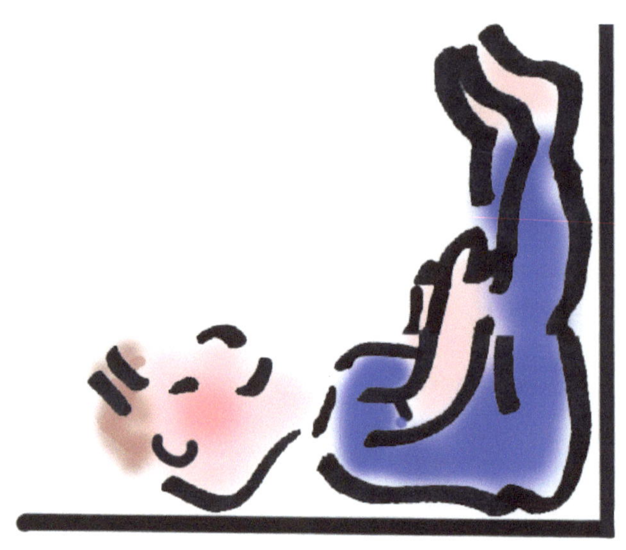

Look at the ceiling and smile.
After a few minutes, squirm away
from the wall and lay down fully.

Are your feet stinky?

Stinky feet spray (water)
will eliminate the smell.

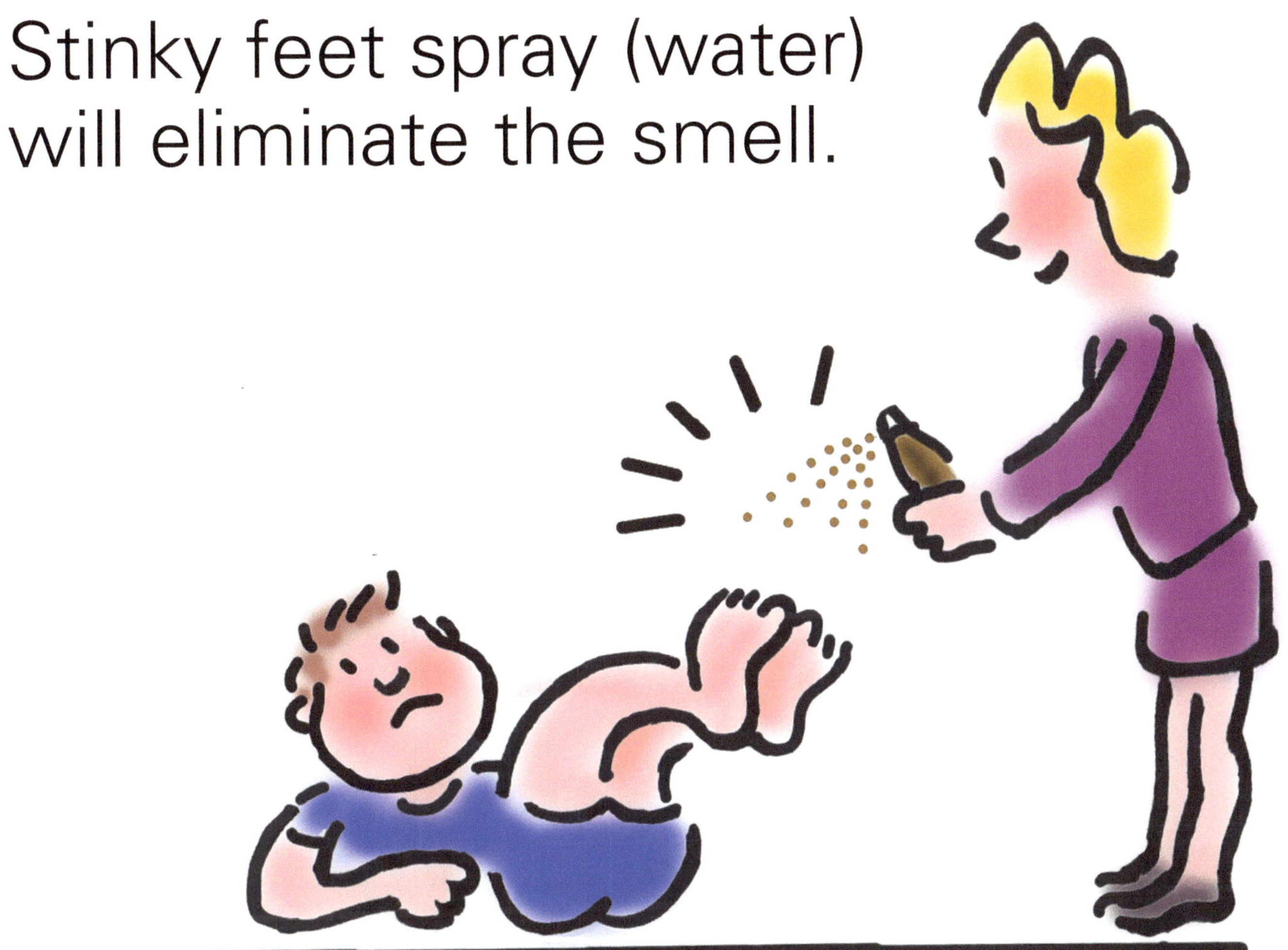

Remain on the ground.

Relax.

Lift your arms in the air, wiggle them, return them to the ground, and relax them.

Lift your legs up in the air, wiggle them, return them to the ground, and relax them.

Fill your belly with air and blow it out.

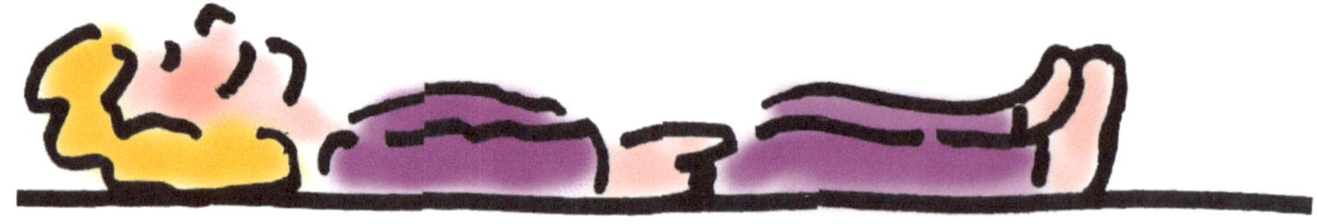

Are you ready for the spaghetti test?

A grown up should be able to pick
up your legs one at a time...

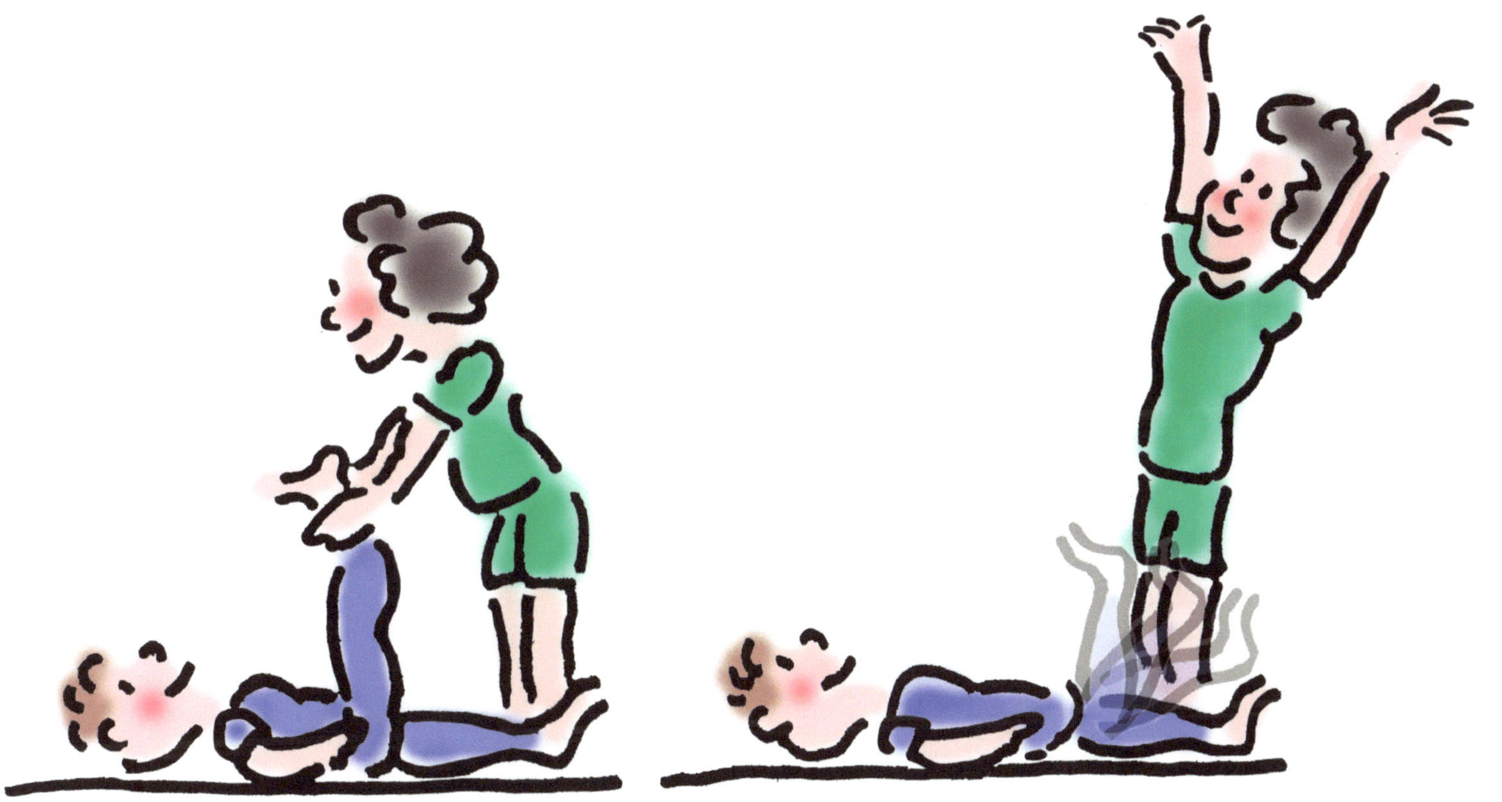

...and when they drop, you should
be so relaxed that they fall like
spaghetti.

Think of your favorite place.
Are there trees or dogs?
Take a moment to stay there
and enjoy.

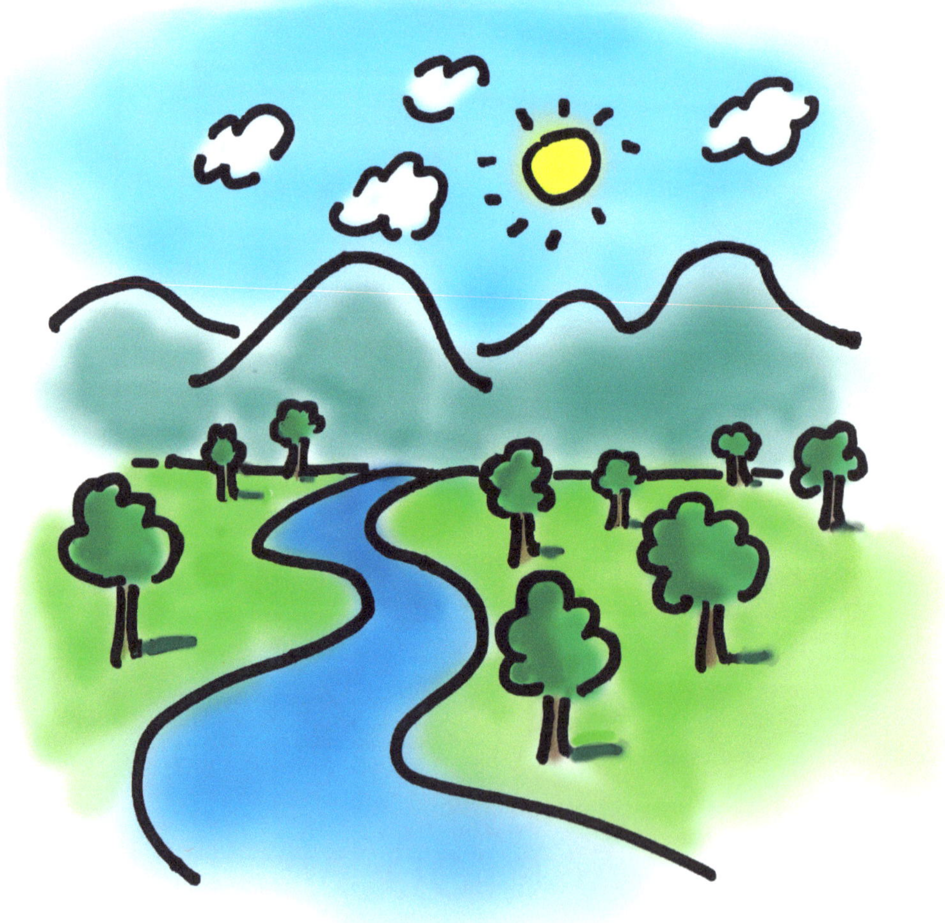

Remember you can always come back to this place whenever you feel like it.

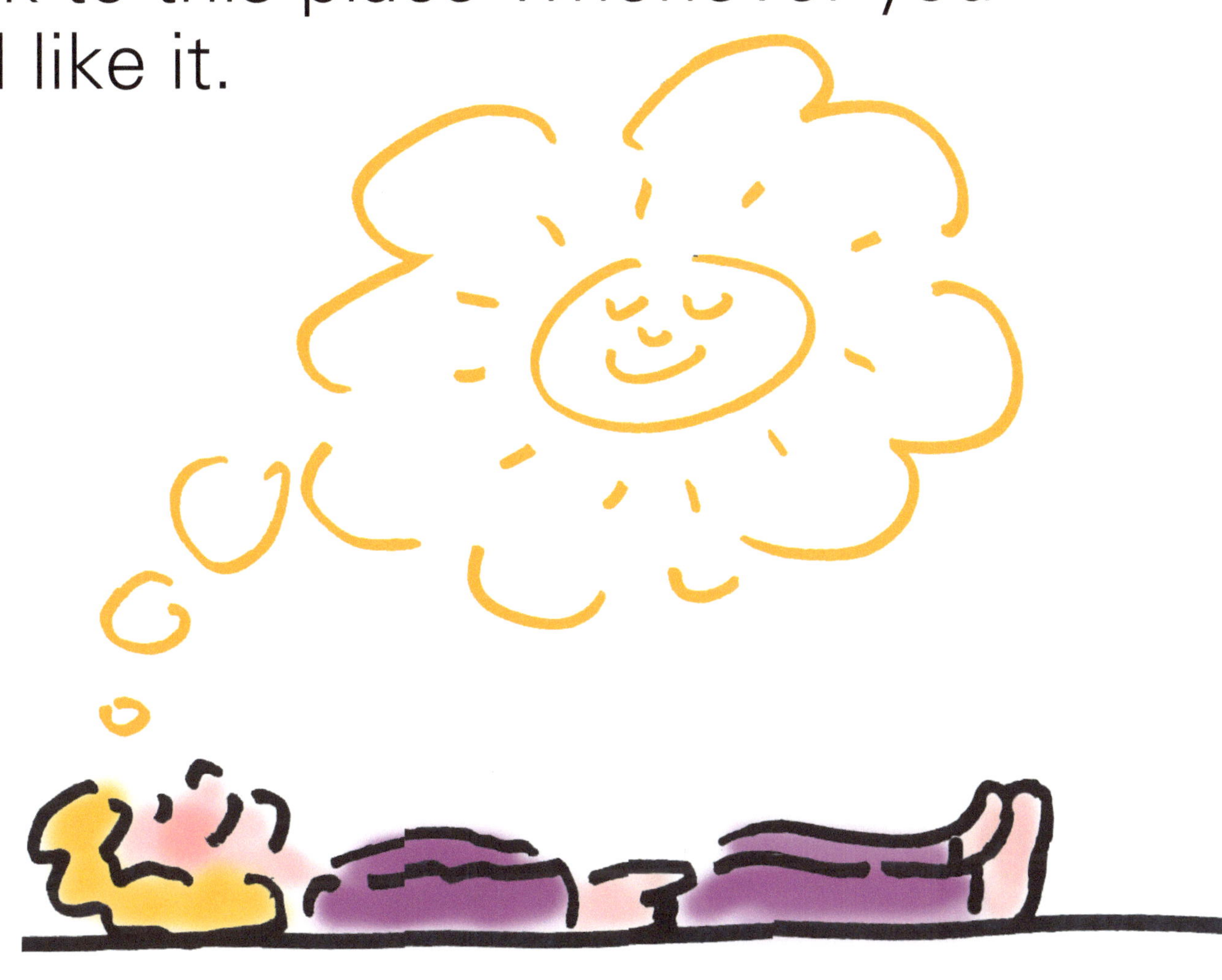

When you are ready, turn to one side and sit up slowly.

Sit in a comfortable seated position one more time. Remember you have many options.
Criss-Cross Applesauce

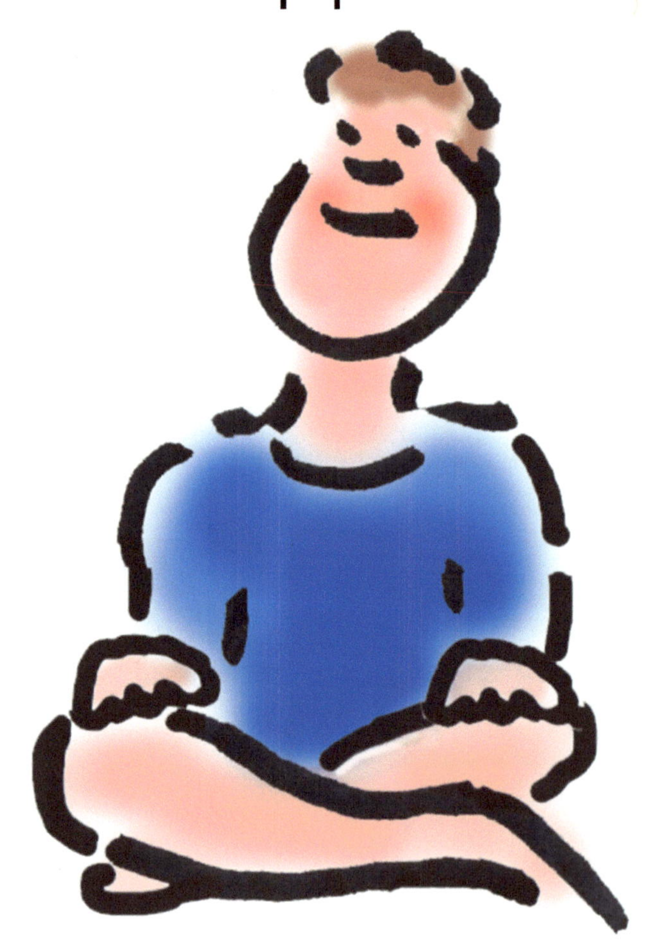

or Half Lotus

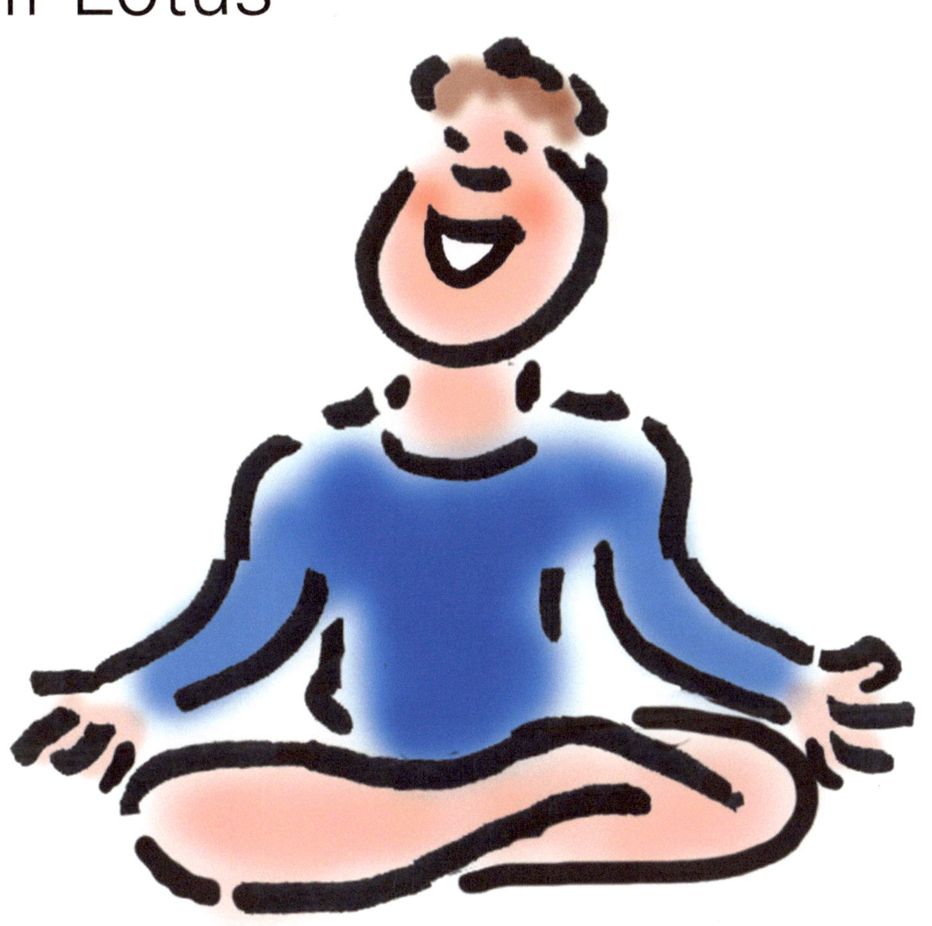

or Full Lotus

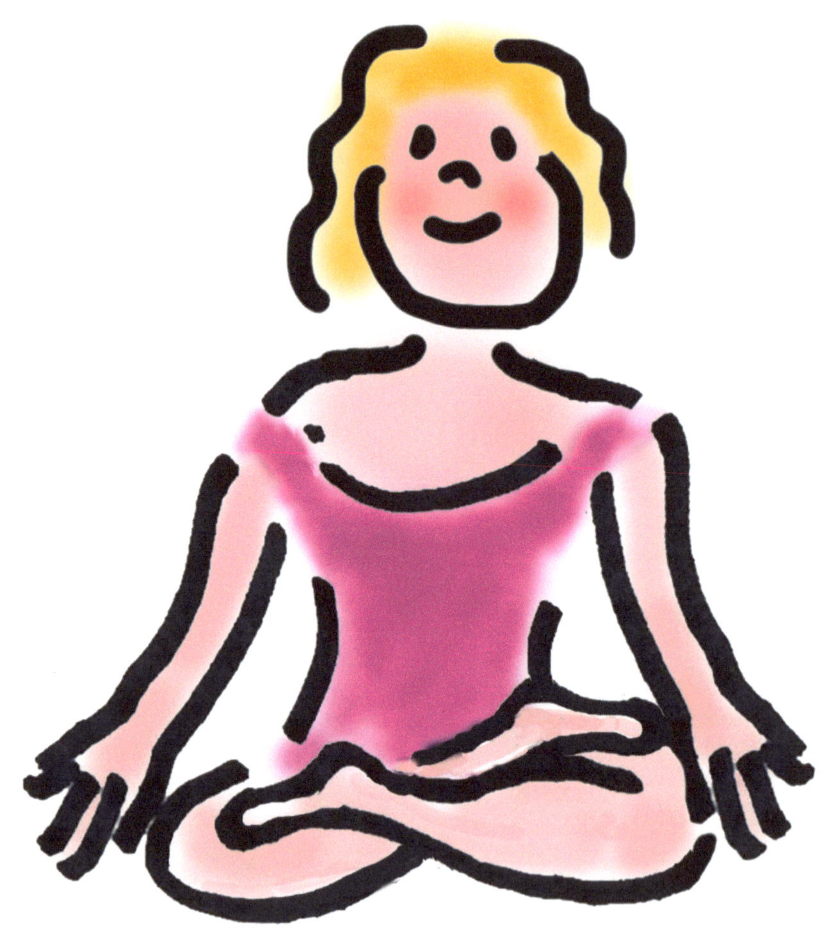

or really however you want

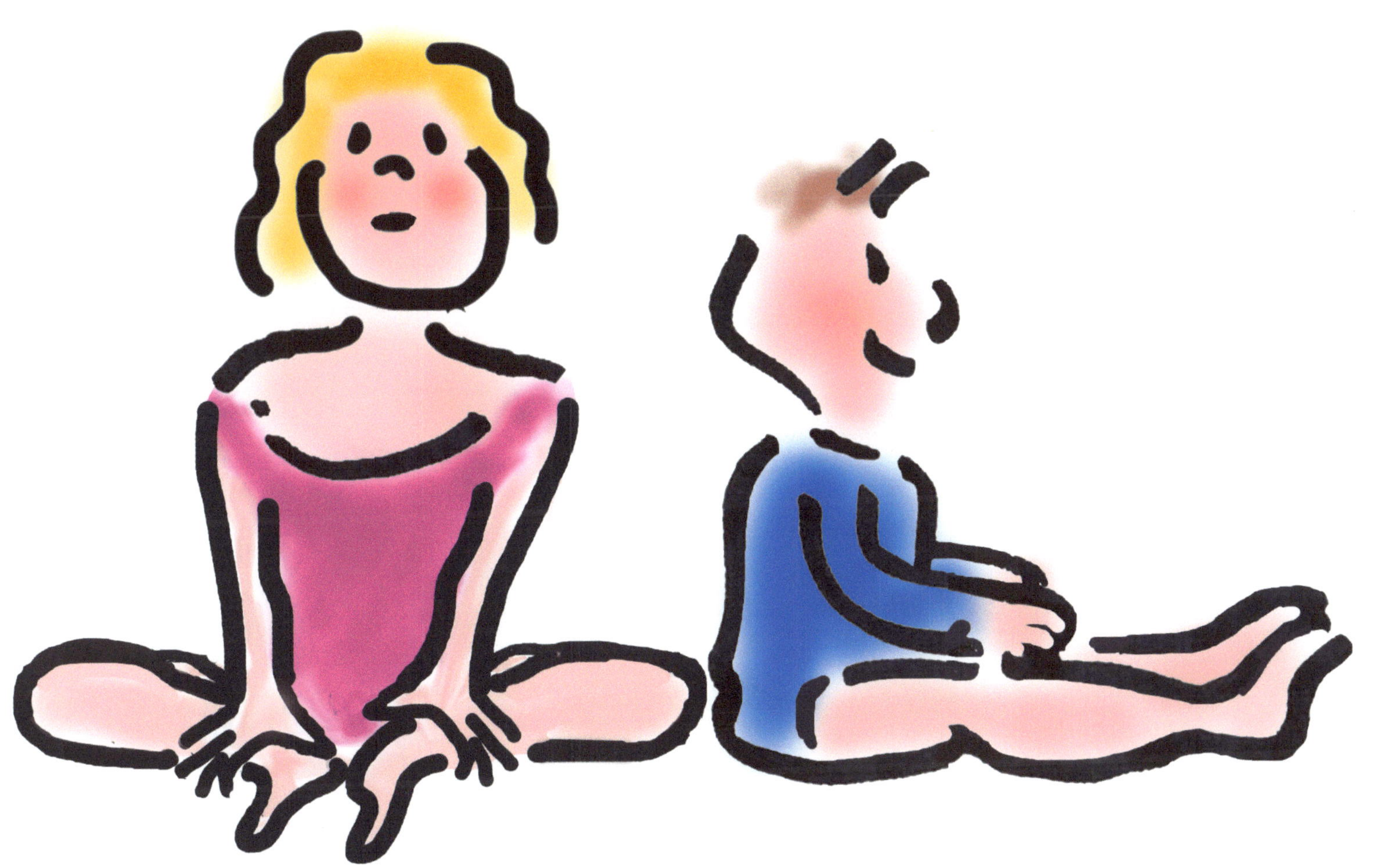

26

Breathe like a bunny!

Take three quick breaths in through the nose

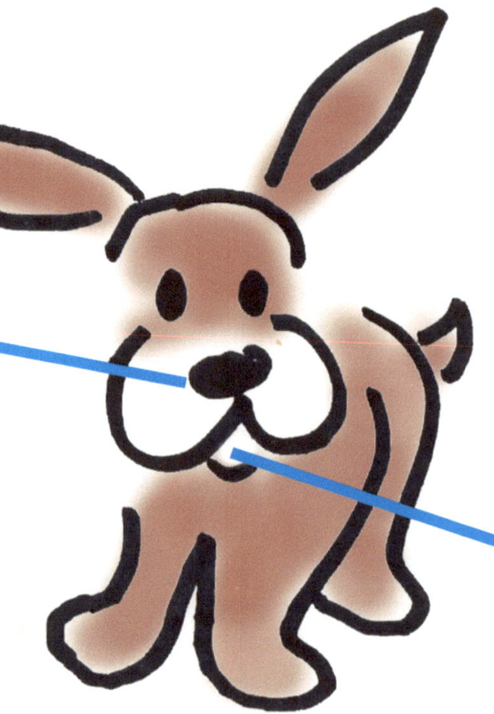

and one out the mouth.

Place your finger on one nostril
and...

then the other.

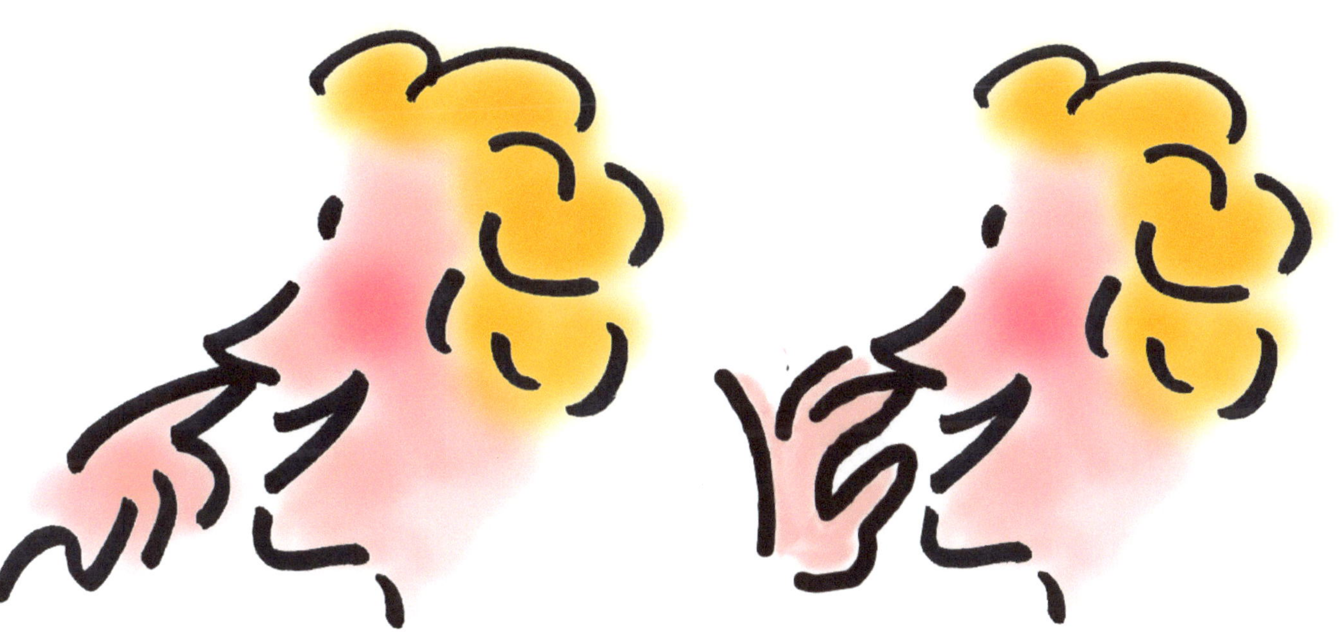

Remember to inhale and exhale
through the opposite unblocked
nostril. Repeat a few times.

Put on your
yoga glasses.

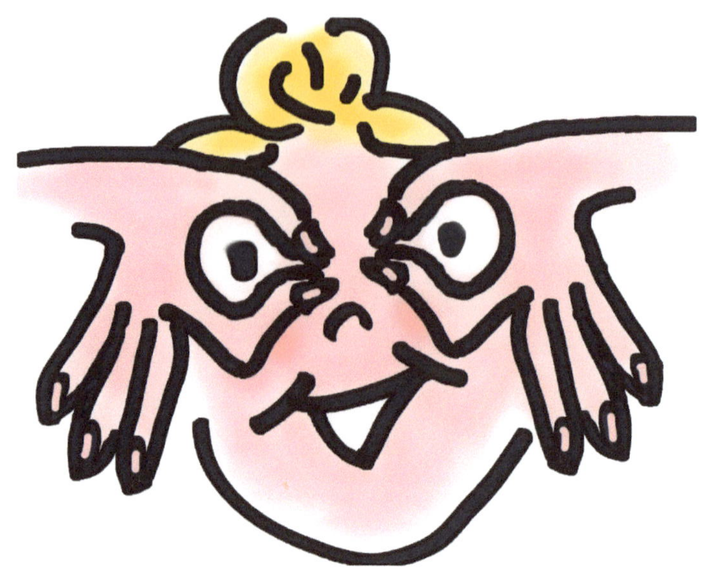

Place your yoga
glasses on your
knees.

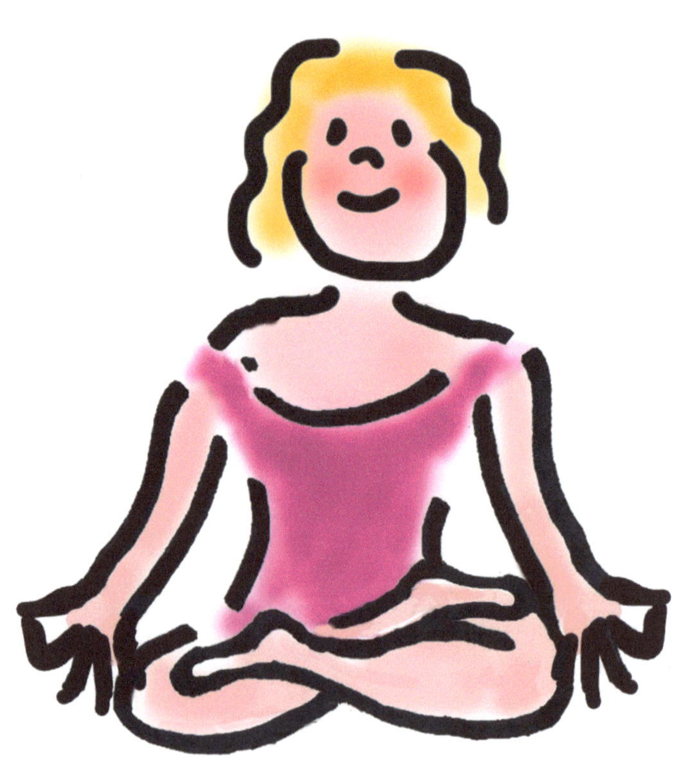

As you touch each finger
to your thumb, say:

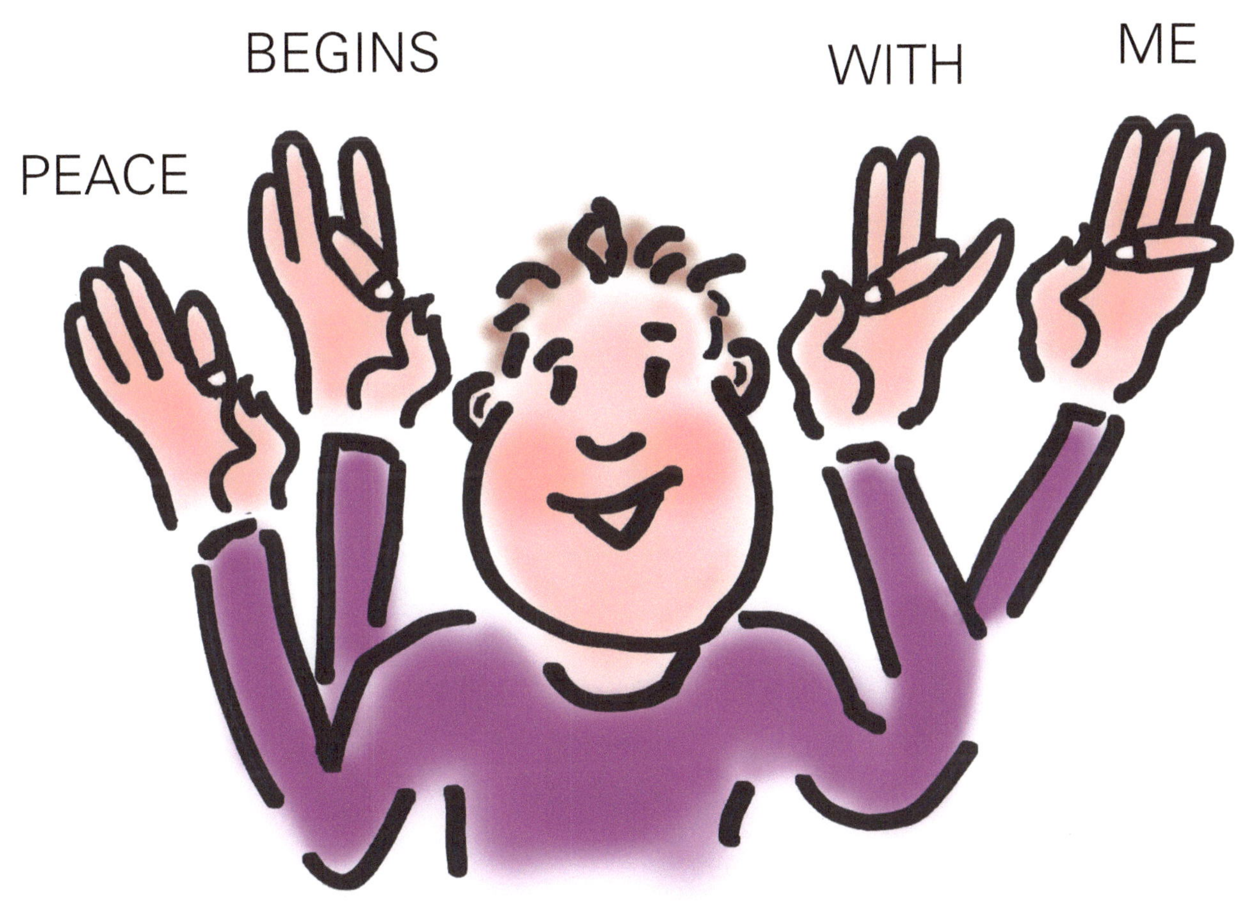

Repeat this phrase quieter each time
until you can only hear it in your head.

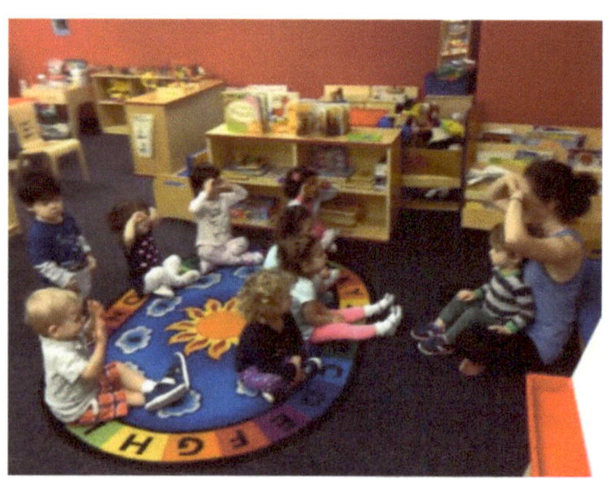

Nina Salpeter is a certified 200-hour, therapeutic, and kids yoga teacher. She lives in New York City with her toddler Max and husband Josh.

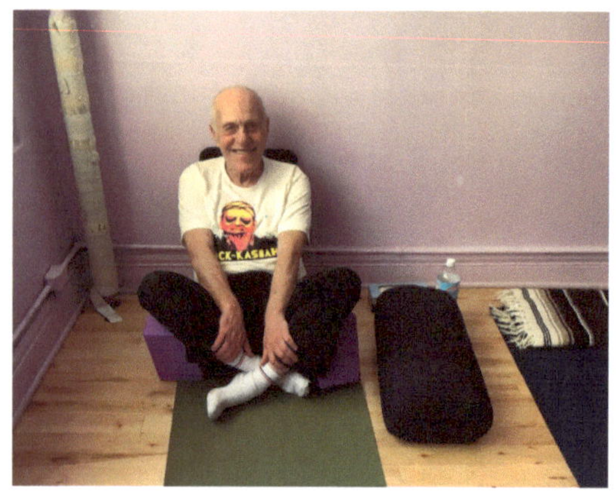

Bob Salpeter has extensive experience in designing corporate and marketing literature, identity programs, advertising, web design, exhibits, and packaging for a wide range of clients. He has received numerous awards from the American Institute of Graphic Art, The Art Director Club of New York, The Type Directors Club, and Design International in Paris, among others.

www.ingramcontent.com/pod-product-compliance
Lightning Source LLC
Chambersburg PA
CBHW040055240726
48664CB00004B/1199